Whole Food:

30 Day Guide to A Healthy Life - Lose Weight, Increase Metabolism & Enjoy Delicious Meals

that the author is not engaging in the rendering of legal, financial, medical or professional advice.

By reading this document, the reader agrees that under no circumstances are we responsible for any losses, direct or indirect, which are incurred as a result of the use of information contained within this document, including, but not limited to, —errors, omissions, or inaccuracies.

Table of Contents

Introduction

A perennially popular topic for discussion worldwide, nothing bonds people like an intense debate on weight loss tips and techniques. People everywhere are desperate to lose weight and keep following fads and diets and yet fail miserably in their quest. So, what exactly is weight loss? It refers to an overall reduction in body mass, be it loss of adipose tissue, water, lean mass, connective tissue or fluids in the body. This can either occur intentionally, through a rigorous weight loss regime, exercise, going to gym, diets or unintentionally, usually signifying a serious medical condition.

People who undergo diets and extreme fads further endanger themselves on account of inadequate and insufficient nutrition. The body has lowered defenses against disease, hormonal changes, fluctuating metabolism and invites a host of parasites and other pathogens for invasion. Unhealthy means of weight loss have always proven to be detrimental in the long run. If you do want to lose weight, do it so gradually and in a healthy manner, with adequate amounts of exercise and a proper diet.

Of course, some people, especially those suffering from weight related problems like obesity, diabetes, back problems etc. need a specific weight loss plan, but that should be done by a licensed nutritionist and fitness trainer. Any intentional weight loss has to be done systematically; otherwise it might induce lasting damage to the body.

Chapter 1: Diets and the Myths Surrounding Them

A diet is basically a planned proportion of food groups that are eaten at periodical intervals of the day. But in order to lose weight fast, say, by the weekend, people go on crash diets and adopt all kinds of fad diets, like eating cotton balls soaked in fruit juice or the juice-only diet or the raw salad diet or the paleo diet. Every day, some new diet appears in the market, endorsed by so-and-so celebrity, and people just blindly follow them, without thinking about the repercussions for a second. A proper diet should include all the major food groups and the number of calories ingested depends on person to person.

For instance, a 110-pound man will have a daily caloric intake of about 1550 calories. This is vastly different from the 180-pound wrestler who needs a special diet and who wants to bulk up. Though the caloric intake differs from person to person, the food being eaten should not skip any of the five major groups- carbohydrates, fats, vitamins, minerals, and protein.

You can eat the most wonderful of combinations in the world, but the extra kilos will continue to pile up unless a formal exercise regimen is followed. You needn't necessarily join the gym in order to lose weight. A simple round of brisk walking will do wonders more than sweating it out in a gym, surrounded by hulks who inevitably judge you. Go for a jog in the mornings, walk the dog, use the stairs, help around in the house, mow the lawn, do simple bodyweight exercises like squats, lunges, push ups and pulls ups.

Whatever you do, be disciplined in your approach. Diet myths abound and it is very easy to fall prey to them. You see your fit-as-a-fiddle neighbor chomp on nothing but carrot and cucumber sticks all day and guzzle copious amounts of lemon water. You might be tempted to do the same, but refrain. Listen to your body.

Ah, your favorite chapter, isn't it? Everywhere you look, in the papers, on the net, on TV advertisements, each day brings forth a new diet plan guaranteed to make your fat disappear and give you a gleaming six pack abs, all by summer. There are so many myths surrounding this particular aspect of health, it's staggering. Here are a few of them. I'm sure you've come across them at some point or the other in your life.

- A low fat, high protein diet is the best of all.
- Eat many small meals, spread throughout the day, to stoke the metabolic flame.
- Do not eat egg yolk, eat only the white. Yolks contain a high percentage of cholesterol, which is bad for the heart.
- Saturated fat is bad for your heart, as it raises the LDL cholesterol.
- Do not drink coffee. It is unhealthy for you and gives you cancer.
- Eating fat makes you fat. Say no to butter, cream, clarified butter, margarine and oil.
- Have skimmed milk and related dairy products. Full fat and full cream dairy raises your cholesterol.
- Low fat foods are better for you, because, well, they contain low calories.
- Do not eat anything after 6 pm.

- Chocolate gives you acne.
- Carbs after 7 pm makes you fat.
- The healthiest diet to follow is low-fat, low carb, high protein with lots of grains.
- Eat several small meals a day, instead of three large meals.
- Avoid eating egg yolks.
- Refrain from eating dairy products, as they are full of fat and unwanted calories.
- Sugar causes diabetes.
- Fasting in the morning can help you lose weight.

If you've raised your hands in recognition to any of these myths, it's time to know that none of this is true. The only way to lose weight in a healthy manner is to eat right, get lots of exercise and an equal amount of rest. Leave the rest to nature, it knows best. Read on to find out which kinds of natural foods will help you in your quest of weight loss, without losing out on the taste factor as well!

Points to keep in mind

1. All diets are not created equal. Some actually need prescribed diets by their physicians to combat obesity and other health related problems.
2. Just because your favorite celebrity endorses a diet is no reason for you to take it up.
3. Use your common sense. Going on a juice-only diet may sound interesting and virtuous even, but your body is screaming out loud for other nutrients. It will soon stop functioning normally if you don't feed it right.

Whole Food

What constitutes a proper diet? What is healthy? Organic food, imported food, exotic sounding food? The answer is simple. What kind of food have you been brought up on? That constitutes your staple diet. Stick to it. Cravings will come and go but your staple diet will never go out of fashion, never get boring and never harm your body. Obviously, steer clear of fried food, street food, anything covered with refined flour and deep-fried. Prepare your own meals at home. Make use of cooking techniques like boiling, broiling, roasting, baking and keep the frying to a minimum.

There's no set diet for anyone. Eat what works for you and do not make drastic changes to your diet. Otherwise it will cause serious repercussions on your body in the long run.

Whew! These are only some of the myths that keep doing the rounds of the Internet and papers. People fall headlong for such untested and unscientific statements made by people who haven't the faintest clue what they're harking on about.

Agreed, a proper diet goes a long way in determining your health. In fact, six packs are not made at the gym; they are made in the kitchen. What you put into your mouth is equally important as what you lift at the gym. If your diet consists of junk food, fried food, foods with empty calories, and apart from the gym or the one hour exercise session at home, you lead a largely sedentary lifestyle, no matter how much you lift or how much time you spend exercising, the results will be disappointing. Studies have shown that people who were active throughout the day, walking here and there, carrying things, climbing stairs, cooking in the kitchen, playing with their children were much healthier on an average than someone who just went to the gym for a couple of hours and sat the whole day. The whole point of exercise and nutrition is to keep your body fit and functioning for a long span of time. Bad eating habits will soon nullify any good that you did at the gym.

Staying Healthy

Almost all nutritionists agree on certain principles for keeping the body healthy and sound.

1. Never Skip Breakfast-

Even if you're hard pressed for time, have a bowl of fruit and milk. Or brown bread with peanut butter. Skipping breakfast will cause hunger pangs later in the day, and you are more likely to munch unhealthy stuff like chips or wafers to combat the hunger. Have a hearty breakfast and watch your energy levels stay up all through the morning.

2. Go Easy on Fast Food-

There's no reason to give up on your favorite pizzas, burgers, fries and tacos. Just make sure you have them in a limited quantity at fixed time intervals. Say, once a month. Even better, make these at home. Then you'll have total control over the ingredients and can make healthier versions of pizzas and burgers right at home.

3. Eat Real Food-

This means food grown in a farm. Whole grains, rice, wheat, maize, corns, millets, beans, pulses, fruits, vegetables, nuts all constitute healthy and whole food. Eating homemade meals made of these will satiate you hunger, fill you with good calories and keep your metabolism active. Anything out of a box is a no-no. Focus on raw ingredients.

4. Drink, drink, drink-

By that, I mean water. Drink as much as you think you need. Forget about the 8-glasses rule or the 5-liter rule. Your body will tell you when it wants food and water. Drink and eat accordingly.

5. Eat Good Fats-

Eating fat won't make you fat. Nuts, butter, avocados all contain good fats that help your joints and muscles function smoothly and not clog your arteries. Eat them in a moderate amount, along with your stir-fries or cereal or just roasted.

Chapter 2: Myths Regarding Diets

Just because your overweight friend decides to go on a diet is no reason for you to follow suit. Diets are primarily meant for people who are grossly overweight or obese, or unhealthy in some way. Getting rid of five to ten percent of bodyweight for an overweight person can work wonders for their body and mind, making their hearts and kidneys healthier. But everywhere we look, we see already healthy people succumbing to this diet fad. Of course, going on a diet has its benefits, but only for people who actually need it.

Advantages of a diet

Weight Loss-

Obviously, the number one reason for embarking on any diet, weight loss not only gives you a pleasing appearance, it helps the body internally as well. Being overweight adds extra strain on your heart, liver, kidneys, joints and it also clogs your arteries. A balanced combination of diet and exercise will work wonders in giving you a whole new life. People put on weight simply because the number of calories they ingest is more than the number of calories they burn, plus a sedentary lifestyle. Instead of crash dieting, eat healthy and get regular exercise.

Lower Blood Pressure-

According to a study published in Diabetes Care, losing between two and five percent of your extra weight will help lower your blood pressure and keep your diabetes under control. Extra weight equals more strain on the heart, and that means higher blood pressure.

Lower Triglycerides-

Triglycerides are important for your body, as they store any extra calories you consume. But constant storage of extra calories is what makes you fat. Higher levels of triglycerides are unhealthy for the heart and may cause coronary problems.

Improved cholesterol and a healthier heart-

A diet may help your good lipids, that is, your high-density lipoprotein (HDL), by boosting your metabolism and keeping your heart active. Plus, reducing your cholesterol levels, your bad lipid levels, increasing your metabolic rate and keeping your blood pressure under normal is vital for a healthy and properly functioning heart, cutting the risk of heart and coronary disease by a large margin.

Lower Glucose Levels-

Losing some weight can aid with the blood sugar levels in the body. This is not only great for diabetics, who can keep a check on their blood glucose levels, but also for anyone who wishes to keep that disease at bay.

Improved Mood and Overall Fitness-

Not only does exercise and weight loss make you look good eventually, you will also begin to feel great and energetic throughout the day. Losing weight and keeping the body fit will result in an overall sense of well being and energy, which no pill or juice can provide.

A diet does have these benefits, but one should be extremely careful about embarking on one. Let's look at some of the most popular and some uncommon diets that are in vogue today. I've not included weird ones like the tapeworm diet or juice only diet or cotton balls dipped in fruit juice diet or the fast food diet. These are just plain stupid. The ones given below are just indicators of what diets are supposed to be like. By no means should you accept a diet just because "everyone is doing it". Consult your doctor, take your individual needs into account and see whether the diet suits you or not.

Types of diets

The world of eating is filled with diets. Every day, someone comes up with a newer and wackier one. Earlier, these diets were religiously followed by movie stars or models and reported in the dailies, which we lapped up with great interest. The past decade has seen a sea change in this attitude. Now, every other person you know is on a diet. The plump little girl who is actually healthy but is constantly overshadowed by her athletic sister, the overworked and tired housewife who is struggling to get back to her pre-pregnancy figure while juggling a baby and other responsibilities, the busy executive who hardly has time for a proper home cooked meal, the friendly grandma at the end of the street who suddenly wishes to lose twenty pounds, the waif-like girl who still needs to fit into a bikini by the end of the week- the list is endless. At any dinner party or an informal gathering, the topic of conversation soon veers off into who is into what kind of diet.

Listed below are some common and ﹘
diets. Let's have a look at them.

The Exchange Diet-

This is one of the better diets to follow
down on any food group and instills
good and healthy eating. It works like this- from each of
the good groups; you are allowed a certain number of
helpings per day. You can include everything-
carbohydrates, fats, protein, vitamins and minerals- but in
a certain quantity. This diet encourages you to eat healthy
and maintain a balance between your body weight-height
ratio. It is one of the best diets to follow because there is no
deprivation involved. You learn to eat wholesome foods
while being in control of the portion sizes.

The Planned Menu Diet-

In this type of a diet, you first make menus for the entire
week, starting from Monday and ending on Saturday.
Sundays can be a cheat day. You get to select what you
want to eat, based on the menu plan. For instance, you
may choose from a predetermined set of breakfast items,
like porridge or bread or cornflakes or pancakes. For
lunches, you choose either lean meats or fish or chicken
and the salads that go with them, plus the method of
cooking. Snacks can comprise of unbuttered popcorn,
carrot sticks, whole-wheat crackers with cheese,
guacamole dip with corn chips etc. So you see, you enjoy
this diet because of its diversity. You don't have to sit and
count your calories at every meal. Just select one or two
food items from each menu and you're done.

Atkins Diet-

There are four phases in this kind of diet:

Phase One- Induction

In this phase, the person eats less than 20 grams of carbs per day for two weeks. Instead, the diet comprises high fat, high protein and green leafy vegetables.

Phase Two- Balancing

This phase sees the person adding nuts, some more vegetables and fruit back into the diet.

Phase Three- Fine Tuning

When the ideal weight loss goal is reached, the person adds more carbs to the diet until the weight loss begins to slow down.

Phase Four- Maintenance

Here, the person has achieved his target goal and can resume his normal diet without worrying about gaining the weight back again.

The Paleo Diet-

This diet aims at eating like we used to back in the olden days. What our caveman brethren used to eat. This includes anything that is available in nature- meat, vegetables, fruits, fish, greens, seeds etc. As a species, somehow we have graduated to eating refined foods, which is the root cause of most of our health related problems. The Paleo diet loads up on meat, vegetables and seasonal produce, instead of bread, pasta, corn, white rice etc. This diet works because this is how we are biologically designed to eat and digest food. The Paleo diet also waves a cheery goodbye to sugar. Unless the sugar comes from a natural source, like a fruit or nut, you can forget about it. Sugar causes your energy systems to spike and crash rapidly, and unused sugar is stored as fat unless used immediately and this causes mayhem in the body. Hence, no sugar. There you have it- no grains, no sugar and no processed foods. Just eat everything available in nature.

The Vegan Diet-

Who is a vegan? Vegetarians are those who do not eat meat, fish or poultry. Vegans go a step beyond this. They do not consume any animal product or by product, such as dairy products, eggs, leather, fur, honey, silk, wool, cosmetics and soaps which are derived from animals and animal products. People choose to turn to veganism for various reasons including health, environmental and ethical. For instance, vegans might argue that by eating eggs and consuming dairy products, we are actually encouraging the meat industry. Makes sense, because when dairy cows or hens or chickens grow too old to lay eggs, they are sold as meat. Male calves have it rough as well. Since they do not produce milk, they are bred for veal or meat or some such purpose. Many people choose to go vegan because of the issues of hygiene and cleanliness in abattoirs and slaughterhouses. Still others adopt this kind of a lifestyle to promote empathy and humanity in their fellow human beings.

Vegan nutrition is actually simple and varied. A typical vegan diet might include lots of fruits, vegetables, green leafy vegetables, whole grains, nuts, seeds, lentils and legumes. If we take protein, it is very easy to find some in the vegan diet as long as the calorie intake is proportionate to body weight. In this diet, there are no strict dietary controls with regards to the calories. Except for alcohol, sugar and fats, almost all the foods in veganism contain some amount of protein. These include- chickpeas, peanut butter, soymilk, broccoli, kale, potatoes, lentils, tofu, spinach, wild rice, whole wheat, and oats etc.

A vegan diet is almost free of cholesterol and saturated fat. Since vegans stick to what is available through plants in nature, it is easy to conform to the safe recommendations with regards to fat. Veganism also promotes a healthy heart and reduces the risk of cancer. You may use foodstuffs like oils, butter, margarine, seed butter, avocado, coconut etc.

Carbohydrates are found aplenty in choices like wild rice, oats, barley, whole wheat, whole quinoa and a special type of rice known as boiled rice.

Weight Watchers Diet-

Quite obviously, in this diet, the aim is to lose the extra pounds first. Therefore, the first two weeks are devoted to eating large helpings of fruits and vegetables, with nuts and seeds, and slowly eliminating fat and carbs from the diet. As the weight slowly regularizes, a normal diet is resumed, but with low quantities of fat and carbohydrates.

Chapter 3: FAQs About Diet and Nutrition

Why do people put on weight?

It's simple. You gain weight because the number of calories you ingest is more than the number you burn. Food is basically fuel that gives energy to your body and this energy content is measured in calories. A slice of bread has about 100 calories and an apple, around 160. Whatever we eat throughout the day keeps adding calories inside our bodies. A person needs to ingest a certain amount of calories per day in order to function properly, and the surplus calories are stored as fat for future use. If not expended, they keep on accumulating and the person gains weight. An example- eating only 50 calories a day more than you will burn will become one pound a year, or close to 30 pounds over three decades. That's weight gain for you.

How do diets work? What is meant by a low fat and low carb diet?

Diets mainly work by restricting your calorie intake. Most people have this image of a diet in their mind- tasteless, bland food made only to sustain oneself. Nothing could be farther from the truth. A diet can be made tasty and filled with wholesome food. Of course, just telling people to eat less won't cut it- they will get hungry and keep cheating. So, all the major diet books and lists do the smart thing by telling people to cut down on "fats" and "carbs" and "no eating after 6 pm". Eliminating one of two food groups will obviously take away a large chunk of calories from one's plate. All major diets try and remove the so-called "fattening foods" from your menu, like potatoes, white rice, bread, pasta, oil etc.

The body basically runs on two kinds of fuels- carbohydrates and fats. Of these two, carbs are used as the primary fuel and fats are stored in case of emergency or kept as reserve. Ounce for ounce, fats contain twice as many calories as the same amount of carbs. Therefore, eating food filled with carbs fills you up with fewer calories, as opposed to foods rich in fats, where smaller quantities are required to fill you up. Taken at face value, fat should make you fat. Which is completely untrue.

Carbohydrates, especially processed ones like white bread, refined flour, pasta, are rapidly converted into glucose and used as energy. The sugar so released triggers a surge in the insulin levels, which in turn causes the blood sugar levels to crash as rapidly as they soared earlier, something which is referred to as a "sugar rush". The brain sends out signals with regards to this low blood sugar and the person feels hungry again. The more we eat foods with empty calories, the more we keep getting hungrier without actually satiating it. And over the years, we put on weight. This cycle can be broken by eating a diet rich in protein and fiber, as they are filled with good calories and keep you satiated for a long time.

Will I be able to sustain my diet for a long-term period?

Sadly, no. Studies have shown that very few people have the will power to stick to a diet. Most of the population enthusiastically begins a diet, feel extremely happy when they begin losing weight through crash dieting and then hit a plateau. From then on, no matter what they restrict in terms of eating or how many hours they spend exercising, the pounds keep piling back on. Disheartened with the results, most people give up and resume their unhealthy eating habits. This is because most diets encourage people to exclude whole food groups. A low carb or low fat diet soon tires the body out which starts demanding food in proper proportions.

Of course, there are people who seem to maintain their weight and stick to a diet for years. Such people are also extremely active than the average dieter. Keeping the extra weight off requires immense discipline and a commitment to lifelong fitness.

Are fats bad for me?

Get this straight. Fats are NOT bad for you. In fact, if you do not feed your body the requisite amount of dietary fats, you will end up suffering from creaky joints, lack luster skin and hair, lack of suppleness in your muscles. Fat is needed to lubricate the joints and muscles of the body and give a glow to your skin and hair. Of course, this does not mean bingeing on fried food every day. Natural fats found in nuts, seeds, oil extracts from nuts and seeds, certain fruits like avocado and olives are good for you and your heart. Cut out the bad fats, like fried food and junk food. Eating fat will not make you fat.

How fat is fat?

It's not a relative term, as is thought. In medical terms, fat or thin is described in terms of your BMI, that is, your Body Mass Index. To calculate your BMI, take your weight (in pounds), multiply it by 703 and divide it by the square of your height (in inches). Anything between 18.5 and 25 is considered normal, between 25 and 30 is overweight and anything above 30 is considered to be obese.

Everyone I know keeps telling me not to eat after 6 pm. Does it make sense?

Absolutely not. All you need to do is ensure that you ingest a certain number of calories each day, depending on your requirement and vital statistics. Roughly speaking, a five-foot tall person weighing about 110 pounds, with a fairly active lifestyle requires about 1500 to 2000 calories per day. Just get that into your body and forget about the 6 pm rule. Of course, it does make sense to eat at the same time every day and get your calories from wholesome foods. Chuck the 6 pm rule out of the window.

Should I eat three big meals or six small meals a day?

Again, it depends on your metabolism and your working habits. If your health and work permit you to enjoy a three-meal-a-day plan, by all means, go for it. If you wish to break your calorie intake into several small meals spread throughout the day, no problem there. It's all about getting your share of the calories for the day.

So, if I'm dieting, I can simply skip breakfast. That will help with the weight loss, right?

Wrong. Absolutely wrong. Skipping breakfast might seem like a good idea in to begin with, but as the morning progresses, you start feeling hungry and cranky, and you will pop into the nearest shop or canteen to buy a candy bar or a bag of chips or some other unhealthy snack and start munching. Skipping breakfast will actually make you gain weight, because you will indulge in mindless eating afterwards. To avoid this, eat a hearty breakfast. After seven hours of sleep, your blood sugar is low in the morning. Feed your body healthy breakfast foods like pancakes, toast, eggs, grits, cereal, milk, coffee etc. Make this a major meal. A hearty breakfast will ensure zero hunger pangs later in the day, plus you will be bursting with energy.

Which is better-an hour of foot and heart thumping aerobic routine or thirty minutes of HIIT or twenty minutes of weight training?

It purely depends on your goals. If your goal is weight loss and keeping your heart strong, a mixture of aerobics and strength training will work. If you wish to get stronger and bigger, along with total body fitness, strength training is the way to. If you cannot afford to go to the gym, bodyweight training is just as effective. Just aim to get enough exercise to keep your heart pumping wildly throughout the routine and keep your body in perfect working order. Eat right, exercise and get plenty of rest. The extra pounds will automatically melt away.

Why are those last five to ten pounds so darn hard to lose?

Most people on a diet see their numbers stop at some point in the program. No matter what they do, the needle doesn't budge from that number. Maybe, you have reached your optimum weight-height balance and do not need to lose any extra pounds. Your body is smart; it will stop losing extra weight when it knows it is in a state of equilibrium.

Chapter 4: Grocery Shopping

Now we come to the heart of the matter. What you buy when you are out shopping for groceries has a direct impact on your diet and eating. It doesn't matter how good and noble your intentions are, if you load your cart with packaged and precooked food, you are doomed even before you've started your diet. Here are a few tips to get you started.

What to Keep in Mind Before You Go Grocery Shopping

Never go to the store with an empty stomach

This is a golden rule to be followed at all costs. Eat something substantial, like a peanut butter sandwich or a protein shake or a fruit salad before you hit the road. If you step inside the store when you're hungry, you will automatically veer towards the aisles containing packaged food items, chips, and candies- anything that will satiate your hunger quickly. So, enter the store with a full stomach. You will make wiser and better choices while buying groceries.

Say goodbye to your favorite "evil" foods-

This means a firm no to refined flours, white sugar, alcohol, trans fat, fried food, packaged meals and instant cook meals.

You don't have to become a kitchen superhero in one day-

Acknowledge the fact that you can't kick your habits of many years. Switching over to clean and healthy foods is more difficult than it seems. Give it some time. Go easy by replacing one or two food items per food group. For example, switch to wheat pasta or soba noodles for the ones made with refined flour. Chuck the Mars Bars and go with dates and figs. Remove white sugar and replace it with honey and jaggery. Add one or two healthy items per shopping trip and as your taste buds get used to them, keep adding to the list. After a while, you will find that the fast food and junk food you used to crave will have lost their appeal.

Less is indeed more-

If something comes in a box with a huge list of ingredients, simply put it back. The more processed a food item is, the less healthy it is. As a rule of thumb, try and avoid eating anything that comes out of a box. Go as natural as possible.

Create your menus with a few food items-

You don't have to buy the entire store's worth of vegetables to create one healthy dish. Mix and match items from various food groups to create simple, tasty and healthy dishes. For instance- you could have honey roasted asparagus with thyme and cilantro for starters, whole wheat pizza with healthy toppings like butternut squash, quinoa, kale, broccoli, onions, bell peppers, jalapeno with a drizzle of olive oil as the main course and a simple, fresh fruit salad with honey for a heavenly dessert.

What to Buy

Let's divide the shopping into different categories like grains, protein, vegetables, fruits, flavorings etc. This will simplify the process.

Grains and Cereals (Carbohydrates)

- ✓ Brown rice
- ✓ Wild rice
- ✓ Wheat
- ✓ Millets
- ✓ Maize
- ✓ Nuts/Seeds (Protein)
- ✓ Quinoa
- ✓ Soba noodles
- ✓ Eggs
- ✓ Beans (different types like kidney, black, cannellini, pinto etc.)
- ✓ Lentils
- ✓ Chickpeas

- ✓ Nuts like almonds, peanuts, groundnuts, walnuts, cashew nuts, dates etc.

- ✓ Sunflower and safflower seeds

- ✓ Vegetables/Herbs/Fruits (Vitamins and Minerals)

- ✓ Generally, one should buy seasonally fresh vegetables, as opposed to canned ones. Buy as many colorful vegetables as possible.

- ✓ Common seasonal produce like tomatoes, potatoes, eggplant, broccoli, sweet potatoes, okra, bottle gourd, bitter gourd, snake gourd, squashes, bell peppers, onions, garlic, spring onions, cabbage, cauliflower, carrots etc.

- ✓ Leafy vegetables like kale, spinach, cilantro, curry leaves, basil, parsley etc.

- ✓ Fruits available locally and seasonally

Condiments/Flavorings

- ✓ Oils like olive, coconut, sunflower, sesame, safflower, and groundnut.

- ✓ Black and cayenne pepper, red pepper flakes

- ✓ Mountain or rock salt

- ✓ Turmeric

- ✓ Mustard or mustard seeds

- ✓ Asafetida

- ✓ Oregano

- ✓ Chili powder or sauce

- ✓ Gomasio

- ✓ Cinnamon

- ✓ Paprika

- ✓ Maple syrup

- ✓ Apple cider and red wine vinegar

- ✓ Miso sauce

Snacks

Don't reach out for that bag of chips. Try these healthier alternatives instead.

- ✓ Hummus with a dip

- ✓ Whole wheat tortillas

- ✓ Dark chocolate

- ✓ Dried coconut chips

- ✓ Quinoa and black bean tortillas

- ✓ Unbuttered popcorn

Beverages

- ✓ Coconut water

- ✓ Kombucha

- ✓ Herbal/soothing teas

- ✓ Milk, including flavored milk

✓ To add to your smoothies, get some berries, chia seeds, cacao powder, and custard powder.

For The Kids

✓ Fresh vegetable or fruit salad with honey

✓ Whole wheat pizza

✓ Frozen fruit smoothies

✓ Whole wheat cookies

✓ Vegetable and fruit sticks

✓ Popcorn

✓ Milk and milkshakes

Chapter 5: Dining Out

So you've stuck to a diet, are exercising every day and generally feel fit and fine. Then you decide to go out and celebrate your promotion at work. Before you know it, you've ingested large quantities of pasta, pizza, burgers or something similar, guzzled alcohol like there's no tomorrow and had a very large portion of tiramisu or chocolate mud pie. What is it about restaurants and fast food joints that derail months of hard work? Why is it so difficult to stick to healthy meal options while dining out? It's easy to be in control of your diet inside the safety of your home. You know exactly what you're cooking. As soon as we hit the road and eat outside, all diet and health plans are somehow tossed out of the window. This section is all about getting a few key points straight in your brain, so that the next time you eat out, you are prepared. Keep these tips in mind to enjoy your meal outside and stay true to your healthy diet plan at the same time.

1.Ask for the dishes "your way"-

Keep your meek and mild behavior at home when you're dining out. It's no place to play coy. Be assertive and ask for the dishes to be prepared your way. If something you want is fried, request for it to be grilled or roasted. If the side order is a mandatory French fries, ask for it to be replaced with a salad instead. Ask for smaller portions of meats and larger portions of salads and vegetables. More often than not, the restaurant will happily oblige you. If it doesn't, consider other dining out options.

2.Ask for the vegetable portions to be increased-

Often, we see only a sprig of parsley or a carved up piece of a carrot or a forkful of squash in the name of "vegetable". Ask for more vegetables to be served and offer to pay extra, if your request is not attended to. Don't be shy about it.

3.Don't go only by the menu-

You have to ask the waiter or the chef how exactly the food was prepared. Don't be misled by the menu. Something that is written as "cholesterol free" might not be fat free or low fat, neither does "light" mean light in calories or fat. Ask and then order accordingly.

4.Be wise when choosing entrees-

Order from the healthy and light section of the entrees, such as soups, crackers, fruit balls, cheese dips etc. Soups are the best option as they are healthy, filling and will stop you from over eating during the main course. If a healthy entree option is not possible, split it with someone. Or if dining alone, ask to box half of your entree.

5.Double your appetizers-

If you're eating out at a place that serves a nice selection of vegetables and seafood, you might want to skip the entree and have two appetizers, instead of one. This will definitely fill you up before you start the main course.

6.Order more salads-

People who eat a large salad before commencing their main meal eat fewer calories on an average than those who don't opt for salads. But remember this- a salad is meant to be healthy. Don't let it turn fatty. To avoid this, say no to creamy sauces or mayonnaise, pasta and potato salads, skip the bacon and fried noodles part. Ask for the salad to be comprised of raw vegetables or boiled or marinated ones, get some fruit added in it, like kiwis, pears or add some nuts to it. For a healthy dressing, ask for some yogurt whipped with honey or fruit puree or some rock salt sprinkled over the salad or even some cheese, like Camembert or feta, which have natural salts in them.

7.Watch your salad add ons-

Even if you're having a raw vegetable salad, if they come loaded with meat or cheese or sauce, you're headed for trouble. A typical Caesar salad served at most restaurants is topped with chicken or shrimp, with plenty of cheese, cream and mayo in the dressing. Fried croutons on the side or top add to the calorie count at a whopping 560 calories. If you want to have salad, have just the vegetables without the frills.

8.Dressing on the side-

The best way to have salad with your favorite dressing without feeling guilty is by having the dressing served on the side. Get it separately in a small bowl; dip your fork into it and then into the salad. You will be surprised to discover how a small amount of dressing makes the salad tastier, plus your salad leaves won't be drenched in oil. This way, you get to enjoy the best of both worlds, without worrying about the calorie intake.

9.Check menus online before you leave-

Most restaurants these days post their menus online, in their sites. They not only tell you what they are serving, but also nutritional information on the food items. This way, you can check which restaurant fits your bill for clean and healthy eating and decide accordingly.

10.Read, and eat between the lines-

Look carefully at the menu choices. Words like crisp, breaded, creamy, stuffed, buttery, pan-fired, au gratin, sautéed etc. are loaded with hidden fats- saturated and trans. Other words and phrases like Parmesan, cheese sauce, wine sauce, scalloped, au lait or au fromage (with dairy products like milk, cheese and ice cream) come loaded with "bad fats". Steer clear of them.

11.Skip the bread basket-

Avoid having bread sticks and various kinds of tempting looking buns from the basket. Ask for a plate of carrot sticks or raw vegetables or fruit balls instead.

12.Your choice of drink-

It would be very wise of you to skip the alcohol, but if you absolutely must, avoid drinks like margaritas, pina coladas, fancy fruit punches etc. They are laced with unwanted sugary calories that only provide taste, no nutrition. Order sparkling water, or a glass of wine, or a light beer or even a simple martini without the extra frills like chocolate liquor or sour apple schnapps or olives.

13.Mix and match-

Indulging in a baked potato? Mix it with some vegetables from the salad bar. Or just ask for some salsa or yogurt dip. Do not venture near the butter and sour cream, that's all.

14.Act fishy, very fishy!

When ordering fish, make sure it's not fried. Instead, go with healthier options like steamed, broiled, baked, blackened, grilled or roasted. If sauces are to be had, ask for them to be served separately, as was the case with salad dressing.

15.Keep drinking water-

Water will help you slow down, enjoy your meal and keep you filled, all the while reassuring your brain that you are eating enough. Once the "full" signal hits the brain, you'll stop eating, even though what you ate was far less than what you are accustomed to.

16.Make an event out of dining out-

If you have to dress up, look nice, book a restaurant, invite friends and family, make sure your kids are on their best behavior, choose a place which caters to everyone and is easy on your pocket- chances are, you might think twice or thrice before deciding to dine out. Make an event out of it. Make a fuss. Don't get casual about eating out otherwise your health will go for a toss.

17.Skip the dessert-

Ooh, that chocolate pudding with raspberry glaze! Or how about the delectable caramel mocha soufflé with a mountain of on top? Or perhaps the divine apple-cinnamon pie, oozing with sugar, syrup and butter? Train your mind to avoid looking at the dessert menu. Go home and eat a fruit salad with honey instead. Or if the craving gets serious, have one or two pieces of dark chocolate. It's much better than digging into sinful desserts at the restaurant and feeling guilty later on.

A Few Ground Rules to Remember

Choose Wisely

While selecting restaurants, you need to keep a few things in mind. Just choosing one randomly won't help you. You need to be careful with your selection if you want your diet and health plan to continue the way it was.

If you are a hardcore seafood eater, it is easier for you to find places that serve fresh catch and sometimes, you also get to see how the fish or prawn or lobster is being cooked.

If steak is more your thing, you have an amazing opportunity to eat high protein (steak) with lots of vegetables. Round it off with a simple, natural dessert and you've just treated yourself to a great meal.

If you are in the mood for Mexican, don't be put off by the myth that all Mexican food is unhealthy. On the contrary, Mexican restaurants serve some incredibly healthy dishes. You should know what you are looking for. Whole-wheat tortillas, salad with salsa or guacamole, pan roasted vegetables in a shimmery chica sauce, black bean burritos- all healthy options you can have.

If Chinese cuisine is more your style, fret not. Have clear soup, spring rolls, vegetables and whole-wheat noodles, broiled chicken in broth, dumplings in clear sauce. Go easy on the hot sauces, though.

If you feel like eating breakfast food, have food like braised bacon and boiled eggs, grits, pancakes with maple syrup, cereal with fruit, a fruit bowl with honey etc.

If fast food makes your mouth water and you're grumpy about not being allowed to eat any of that, do not worry. Just choose healthier options. Instead of French fries, have baked potato wedges. Replace the pizza base with one made of whole wheat. Choose healthy toppings like vegetables, lean meats, use cheese sparingly and instead sprinkle lots of herbs and seasoning.

Let the Waiter Become Your Friend

Get out of your comfort zone and speak up. Talk to the waiter/waitress, talk to the chefs and get healthy food items on your plate. Being coy might earn you brownie points elsewhere; this is not the place for that. If you get a plate of chicken sandwich or a burger, have it replaced with lean meat and vegetables. Most of the time, restaurants will oblige customers with custom made dishes which are obviously, not too difficult to plate up.

Say Goodbye to Starch

The starter section at any restaurant is similar- most of the will have a protein/starch/carb option, such as steak and potatoes, fish and rice, cheese and olives etc. A separate vegetable section is also present in some, with veggies like asparagus, greens, kale, spinach etc. If you follow a Paleo diet, replace the starch/carb option with more vegetables that are either grilled or roasted or broiled. If you want to stay safe, just order two helpings of vegetables. If you are not on a Paleo diet but still wish to eat healthier, replace the regular potatoes with sweet potatoes. They are much more filling due to their high fiber content. If you must have fries, have baked or roasted potato wedges and sprinkle some seasoning and herbs on them, instead of cheese or butter.

Salad to Salad

Be careful while ordering salads at restaurants. Though it might seem like a healthy option to us, restaurants often serve salads with the dressing poured over them. The dressing is most often a combination of mayo or cheese or oil or a cream sauce. Have your dressing brought separately and check the contents of the salad. The vegetables and fruits should be as natural as possible, not oozing oil and cream.

Desert the Dessert

There is a truckload of a difference between homemade desserts and restaurant desserts. You know exactly what you are putting into your cakes or pies or puddings or trifles or soufflés. Not so outside. The portion sizes are huge for a single person and we give in to our temptation, only to regret the decision later on. Train yourself not to look at the dessert menu at all. Instead, go home and eat some fruit or make a fruit tart with a honey glaze or simply have a small bowl of ice cream with nuts or some dark chocolate sauce. If you are with friends and everyone else is enjoying their dessert, sip some hot coffee or ask for hot chocolate. If possible, split your portion of dessert and share it with someone. It goes for the entree and appetizer as well. If you feel you cannot finish it yourself or if the portions are too big for you, share it with your tablemates. Enjoyment is possible without stuffing your face and feeling guilty afterwards.

Water, Water, Everywhere

Drink plain or sparkling water, instead of soda, juices or other sugary drinks. Steer clear of alcohol if you know you won't be able to control yourself. If you can, limit it to one glass of wine or light beer. The best option is water, followed by unsweetened lemon water, or lemon water with honey, or iced tea or herbal tea.

Eating While Traveling

Travel somehow makes us all very hungry indeed. Out plop open the bags of chips and pretzels and candy bars. Stop this habit. Load your car with healthy snacks like wheat biscuits, whole meal corn chips, banana fritters, popcorn, dark chocolate, peanut butter bars, granola bars, vegetable sticks, fruit and lots of water. Also, when eating at food joints and motels, look for options that are grilled or broiled or baked or roasted.

Eat Slowly

Enjoy and savor each bite of your food. It takes a full minute for your brain to realize that the stomach is full and satiated. You don't know how much you're stuffing inside yourself when eating in a hurry. So, slow down and let your brain come to the conclusion that your stomach is full.

Resort to Excuses!

Harmless, of course. If you are with a group of people who just won't agree to the fact that you won't eat dessert or won't have another helping of fried shrimp or chicken, just tell them that you have an allergy to those food items. They will stop pushing you and you get to eat what you want, without hurting anybody.

Leftovers Are Okay

In certain cultures and traditions of the world, it is considered rather rude to leave food on one's plate. While that is understandable in a home environment, to clear your plate at a restaurant seems daunting, what with the portion sizes and spices used. If you cannot clean your plate, leave it be. If you are worried about wasting food and feel guilty about it, just have it boxed for you to take home.

Chapter 6: Kitchen Essentials

So, you're all set with great intentions to begin a new, healthy diet. You step into your kitchen, bursting with energy and pumped up about wanting to make a delicious baked chicken breast with a delicate thyme and basil seasoning with some honey glaze. You curse yourself as you look around the kitchen, and find nothing but plastic spoons and empty take away cartons. There's no pan in which you cannot bake and simmer your sauce in, no ladle to stir it, no pots of seasoning on the shelf either, no equipment for carefully julienning the vegetables, nor do you have a peeler or a grater. Frustrated and dejected, you crumple the recipe and head straight to Pizza Hut.

You must have certain kitchen essentials before embarking on a healthy cooking journey. It is maddening to get halfway through a complicated recipe and chuck it all out just because you don't have a measuring cup for the flour. It's time to stop using your cookbooks as coasters and balance your wobbly tables with. Whether you are stocking your kitchen supplies for the first time or looking for a complete overhaul, take a look at the list given below and start entertaining like a pro!

A Set of Knives

A proper set of knives, sharp and functional, is vital for proper chopping and dicing. Look for knives with a stainless steel body so you won't have to worry about them getting rusty. Also, keep cleaning your knives with warm water periodically so they remain clean and shiny.

Cutting Board

A good quality cutting board is extremely important to streamline your cutting, chopping and dicing. While the plastic ones are inexpensive and easily available, look for wooden boards. These are sturdier and keep germs away for a longer time. Some cutting boards come with the cutters attached to them, but be careful about using them. The cutters tend to swing wildly if you are not on the lookout.

Measuring Cups and Spoons

These are of course, invaluable for baking, but also otherwise. Measuring rice and lentils, for instance, or for putting in spices, herbs and seasoning in your dishes, these cups and spoons are a handy aid in the kitchen.

Scissors and Shears

Two very useful tools in the kitchen, these are always getting misplaced. Shears in particular are useful for chopping, slicing, dicing and cutting vegetables, fruits and even meat.

Colander

When you want to drain your pasta or noodles, or while cleaning vegetables and greens, a colander is a boon in the kitchen. No more messy pot lids and pans, with the danger of the produce or food item running away with the water.

All you need is a colander and you're good to go in this department.

Can Opener

Imagine staring at a can of delicious peas or pineapple or coconut milk and lamenting because you do not have an opener. How terrible! Get one and hang it at eye level somewhere in your kitchen. You'll always thank you stars for this.

Mixing Bowls

Think they are only used for mixing stuff? Think again. You can use the bowls for marinating meat, dressing your vegetables, make sauces, dips, and salad dressings and even for dessert. Get yourself a set of bowls, which usually come nested- smaller ones within the larger ones. Get them in stainless steel; they're much better than the pretty but fragile glass ones.

Blender

This can either be a hand blender or an electric one, depending on your budget. Blenders are used to whip up smoothies, drinks, nut butters, sauces, buttermilk, and milkshakes and just about anything that needs to be blended. A blender certainly makes life easier.

Grater

You must have only known or used a grater for grating cheese, but it can be used for besting citrus fruits such as lemon and orange, shredding chocolate into strips, vegetables like potatoes, zucchini and carrots into various shapes. A must have in the kitchen.

A Wire Whisk

A wire whisk is mostly associated with beating eggs, but it has other uses as well. It's great for whipping cream, making sauces, mixing vinaigrettes, removing lumps from gravies and custards, homogenize baking ingredients and scraping off the bits attached to the pan during cooking.

A Vegetable Peeler

Usually, you just peel your vegetables using a knife, ending up with more vegetable on the peel than in your dish. Use a peeler instead; it's practically foolproof and accident proof. You get to save your fingers, at the same time peel off ribbons magically from carrots and potatoes and gourds. A vegetable peeler can also be used to shave off hard cheeses like Parmesan and Gouda, and also for getting chocolate ribbons out of chocolate blocks.

A Pair of Tongs

An invaluable kitchen aid, a pair of tongs can save your fingers from being burnt. Use them for tossing salads, stir-fries, flip your meats or even squeezing juice out of lemons. Sometimes, in cases of emergency, they can also be used as a bottle opener!

A Rolling Pin with Board

After you've made your dough for pies or biscuits or pizzas, you need a rolling pin to roll them out perfectly. When you choose a pin, take one which is longer than the area of the rolled out dough to ensure that the rolling is even. If you take one that is shorter, you will have to roll one area, then go on to the next one, and the result might be uneven.

Saucepans

Saucepans are not used only for making sauces in; they are used for a multitude of purposes. Boiling milk, simmering soups, cooking grits, making Spanish omelets, blanching greens, making tea- a saucepan will come to your rescue most of the time.

Ladles

You will need ladles and spoons of all sizes. Whether you are cooking a curry or flipping pancakes or making soup or creating the perfect pie, you will need ladles and spoons. Get some wooden ones and some in stainless steel.

Spatula

A spatula is a godsend for scrambling eggs, stirring sauces, flipping pancakes and scraping the pan out after cooking. Look for silicone-coated models that are long lasting and have greater heat resistance.

Sauté Pan

Now, this is different from a regular saucepan and a skillet. A sauté pan has straight sides and are perfect for cooking greens, making soups and braising meat. You will not spill any sauce or liquid if you use this pan.

Skillet

Another versatile and invaluable kitchen tool, a skillet can be used for cooking almost everything. There are non-stick varieties available as well, where with a smidgen of oil, you can cook your dish without any further guilt, as no extra butter or oil is required to lubricate it. If you wish to use a cast iron skillet, be sure to keep cleaning it regularly, otherwise it may accumulate rust and germs over a period of time.

A Baking Sheet

Even if you don't bake now, a baking sheet comes in handy for other things. You can use it to make fries, roast veggies, cook chicken and bacon, dry roast spices etc. It is super easy to clean as well. Before you cook, cover the surface with aluminum foil and some cooking spray. After you are done with everything, discard the foil. You don't need to wash the sheet very often either.

An Oven/Microwave Combination

A great piece of equipment to have, even when you don't bake that often. Use it to heat things up, or make slow roasted meals like a pot roast or chicken potpie, even soups. Of course, when you begin baking, an oven will magically turn your dough and batter into mouth-watering cakes, pies, puddings and tarts.

Oven Mitts, Baking Pans and Bowls

Now, obviously, if you have an oven, you need oven mitts and the various dishes and pans that go with it. Keep two sets of the mitts handy. There are specific instructions on the baking pans and bowls with regards to temperatures, material that can be used in the oven. Pay heed to those instructions else you will end up with burnt vessels or worse.

Roasting Pan

Primarily intended as a tool for roasting and braising meat, this kind of pan can also be used to make meat loaves, casseroles, lasagna, rolls etc. The result is quite juicy and succulent. If you buy one with a rack or a grill, you can even cook some yummy Thanksgiving turkey!

Cooling Rack

It is an extremely important element in any kitchen, which will help cool your cookies and pies and biscuits quickly, evenly and keeps them crisp.

Strainer

A tea strainer! Do not forget to include this in your shopping list. You are ready with your lovely, scented herbal tea and discover, to your utter dismay, that you do not possess a strainer. Get one in stainless steel.

Rice Cooker

An invaluable equipment when you wish to cook rice in a jiffy. Just plop in the ingredients into the cooker, sauté them nicely till they release their aroma, put in some spices and condiments, perhaps some vegetables and lentils as well, to make it even more wholesome. Measure out the rice and mix it nicely with the rest of the ingredients. Pour in two and a half cups of water, close the lid and wait for the cooker to work its magic! You will be rewarded with a fragrant rice dish with vegetables.

Chapter 7: Meal Plans

This is a sample diet plan given for ten days. You may mix and match according to your taste and mood. Let's take a look at the plan, shall we?

Day 1:

- ✓ Breakfast: Open egg sandwich, low fat milk, oats

- ✓ Lunch: Turkey pecan salad with vinegar and balsamic dressing

- ✓ Snack: Pear or carrot sticks

- ✓ Dinner: Chicken stir fry with brown rice

- ✓ Dessert: Dark chocolate or an orange

Day 2:

- ✓ Breakfast-Oats, fat free milk, walnuts, raisins and grapefruit

- ✓ Lunch-Chicken soup with cilantro, salad

- ✓ Snack-Peach and tea

- ✓ Dinner-Steak and mushrooms

- ✓ Dessert-Low calorie fudge bar or peanut butter bar

Day 3:

- ✓ Breakfast-Flax meal, bananas, fat free milk, whey protein

- ✓ Lunch-Open face tuna sandwich, salad, cherries

- ✓ Snack-Berries

- ✓ Dinner-Skinny chicken stir fry with wheat spaghetti

- ✓ Dessert-Vanilla ice milk with almonds and walnuts

Day 4:

- ✓ Breakfast-Spanish omelets with shredded Jack cheese, coffee with low fat milk

- ✓ Lunch-Turkey slaw wrap with olives

- ✓ Snack-Hummus and herbal tea

- ✓ Dinner-Green Island shrimp/stir fried shrimp with salad

- ✓ Dessert-Dark chocolate or marshmallows with herbal tea

Day Five:

- ✓ Breakfast-Yogurt with low fat granola, a cup of strawberries and blueberries with almonds

- ✓ Lunch-Grilled chicken and salad

- ✓ Snack-Whole wheat roll

- ✓ Dinner-Asian tuna (broiled) with soba noodles and cashews

- ✓ Dessert-Graham crackers with low fat cream cheese and an apple

Day Six:

- ✓ Breakfast-Homemade pancakes with raspberries and yogurt

- ✓ Lunch-Grilled vegetables and feta cheese wrap

- ✓ Snack-Almonds and herbal tea

- ✓ Dinner-Pepper and cinnamon steak with potatoes and grilled asparagus

- ✓ Dessert-Oatmeal cookies with mozzarella cheese

Day Seven:

- ✓ Breakfast-Whole wheat bagels with cream cheese and salmon

- ✓ Lunch-Bean soup with carrots and walnuts

- ✓ Snack-Whole grain roll with herbal tea

- ✓ Dinner-Vegetarian lasagna with basil

- ✓ Dessert-Vanilla ice milk with almonds and cherries

Day Eight:

- ✓ Breakfast-High fiber cereal with low fat milk and strawberries

- ✓ Lunch-Curried turkey wrap with yogurt and cucumber

- ✓ Snack-Whole wheat biscuits with almonds

- ✓ Dinner-Spic shrimp in wild rice with black beans and lemon

- ✓ Dessert-Dark chocolate with an orange

Day Nine:

- ✓ Breakfast-Two hard boiled or soft boiled eggs with whole wheat toast and honey

- ✓ Lunch-Tuna salad with asparagus, chives and anchovies

- ✓ Snack-Walnuts and a peanut butter bar

- ✓ Dinner-Roasted chicken cutlets with grilled vegetables and balsamic vinegar

- ✓ Dessert-Low calorie fudge bar with unsalted peanuts or yogurt and blueberries

Day Ten:

- ✓ Breakfast-Yogurt, bananas, walnuts and ground flaxseed with coffee

- ✓ Lunch-Chicken salad with salad greens, mushrooms, celery and basil.

- ✓ Snack-Whole wheat roll with herbal tea

- ✓ Dinner-Lemon chicken with olive oil, cabbage, lemon juice, and whole grain pasta.

- ✓ Dessert-Vanilla ice milk with chocolate syrup and almonds or pistachios

Do not fall prey to the diet fads cropping up every day. Listen to your body; it is smarter than you think it is. Feed it good, wholesome food and exercise daily. You will remain healthy for a long time.

Your body is the only place you have to live in. Make it beautiful. Make it healthy. Start now.

Chapter 8: Whole foods Breakfast Recipes

Breakfast Quinoa

Ingredients:

- 1 cup quinoa
- 2 cups water
- 1/4 teaspoon salt

To serve:

- 1 cup berries of your choice or fresh fruits, chopped
- 1 cup rolled oats
- 1/4 cup almonds, sliced
- 1/4 cup pumpkin seeds
- Honey to taste
- Almond milk as required

Method:

1. Place a saucepan over medium heat. Add quinoa, salt and water. Mix well. Bring to a boil.
2. Reduce heat, cover and cook until done.
3. Add the toppings, and serve.

Mexican Potato Omelet

Ingredients:

- 6 large eggs, well beaten
- 1 1/2 tablespoons olive oil, divided
- 1 red potato (4-5 ounces), rinsed, scrubbed, halved, thinly sliced
- 2 cloves garlic, finely chopped
- 1 cup tomatoes, chopped
- 2 green onions, thinly chopped
- 1/4 teaspoon sea salt or to taste
- 1/4 teaspoon pepper powder or to taste
- 1/3 cup pepper Jack cheese
- 2 tablespoons fresh cilantro, chopped
- 1/2 teaspoon fresh lime juice

Method:

1. Add half the oil to a broiler proof skillet and place over medium low heat.
2. Add potatoes, cover and cook until golden brown. Stir occasionally. Add garlic, most of the scallions, salt and pepper and sauté for about a minute.
3. Add the remaining oil to the pan.
4. Meanwhile, add 1/4-cup tomatoes and 1/4-cup cheese to the eggs and mix well. Pour over the potatoes and cook until the center is almost done.
5. Sprinkle remaining tomatoes, scallions, cilantro, lime juice and cheese over it.
6. Broil in a preheated broiler for 2-3 minutes.
7. Cut into wedges and serve with salsa.

Poached Eggs Over Collard Greens & Shiitake Mushrooms

Ingredients:

- 6 large eggs
- 9 fresh shiitake mushrooms, thickly sliced
- 9 cups collard greens, chopped
- 1 large onion, halved, thinly sliced
- 1 1/2 tablespoons apple cider vinegar
- 5-6 cups water
  Dressing:
- 1 1/2 tablespoons fresh ginger, minced
- 5 cloves garlic, pressed
- 1 1/2 tablespoons fresh lemon juice
- 1 1/2 tablespoons extra virgin olive oil
- 1 1/2 tablespoons soy sauce
- 1/4 teaspoon white pepper powder or to taste
- 1/4 teaspoon salt or to taste

Method:

1. Pour water and vinegar to a large shallow pan and place over high heat. Bring to a boil.
2. Lower heat, add eggs and cook until done.
3. Meanwhile, steam together collard greens, mushrooms and onions for about 5 minutes.
4. Mix together all the ingredients of the dressing in a small bowl and set aside.
5. Pour dressing over the steamed vegetables and toss well. Transfer on to individual plates. Place poached eggs over it and serve.

Whole Wheat Buttermilk Pancakes

Ingredients:

- 2 cups whole wheat flour
- 4 tablespoons brown sugar
- 1/4 teaspoon cooking soda
- 2 cups buttermilk
- 1 teaspoon baking powder
- 1/4 teaspoon salt
- Cooking spray
- Honey to serve
- Berries to serve

Method:

1. Mix together all the dry ingredients in a bowl. Pour buttermilk and whisk well until it is free from lumps. Set aside for 10-15 minutes.
2. Place a nonstick skillet over medium heat. Spray with cooking spray. Pour about a ladle of batter. (Pour according to the size of pancakes you desire). Swirl the pan so that it spreads a little.
3. Bubbles will start appearing on the top of the pancake. Cook until the underside is golden brown (or the color you desire). Flip sides and cook the other side too.
4. Repeat step 2 and 3 with the remaining batter.
5. Top with honey and serve with berries.

Breakfast Bagel

Ingredients:

- 2 large eggs
- 1 whole wheat bagel, halved, toasted
- 4 slices tomatoes
- 4 slices avocado
- 4 ounce low fat cheese
- 2 teaspoons apple cider vinegar
- Salt to taste
- Pepper powder to taste

Method:

1. Pour water and vinegar to a large shallow pan and place over high heat. Bring to a boil.
2. Lower heat and add eggs and cook until done.
3. Place 2 slices tomatoes and 2 slices avocado on each half of toasted bagel. Sprinkle cheese over it. Place an egg each over the cheese. Sprinkle salt and pepper and serve.

Chapter 9: Dips n Dressings

Salsa

Ingredients:

- 4 ripe tomatoes, deseeded, finely chopped
- 8 cloves garlic, minced
- 1 cup onions, minced
- 1 small green bell pepper, finely chopped
- 2 cans (4 ounce each) jalapeno pepper, diced or to taste
- 2 tablespoons fresh ginger, minced
- 1/2 cup fresh cilantro, chopped
- 4 tablespoons lemon juice
- 2 tablespoons extra virgin olive oil
- Salt to taste
- Pepper powder to taste
- 1/2 teaspoon cumin powder

Method:

1. Mix together all the ingredients in a bowl and set aside for a while for the flavors to set in.
2. It can last for 4-5 days if refrigerated.

Hummus

Ingredients:

- 3 cups well-cooked chickpeas preferably home cooked, drained but retain some of the drained liquid.
- 3 cloves garlic, peeled
- 1/3 cup extra virgin olive oil +extra for top
- 1 tablespoon paprika or to taste
- 1/2 tablespoon ground cumin
- Juice of 2 lemons
- 3/4 cup tahini with its oil (optional)

Method:

1. Add all the ingredients except parsley to the food processer and blend until smooth.
2. Transfer into a bowl. Drizzle some olive oil. Sprinkle some more cumin, paprika and parsley. Fold gently and serve.
3. Refrigerate the unused hummus. It can last 4-5 days if refrigerated.

Thai Peanut Sauce

Ingredients:

- 2/3 cup unsalted creamy peanut butter
- 1/2 cup soy sauce or tamari or coconut aminos
- 1/2 cup orange juice
- 2 teaspoons red pepper flakes
- 2 cloves garlic, minced (optional)

Method:

1. Whisk together all the ingredients until smooth.
2. Transfer into an airtight container and refrigerate until use.

Honey Mustard Dressing

Ingredients

- 1 cup plain Greek yogurt
- 3 tablespoons honey
- 2 tablespoons lemon juice
- 4 tablespoons yellow mustard

Method:

1. Add all the ingredients to a bowl. Whisk well and use.

Italian Herb Dressing

Ingredients:

- 1/2 cup white wine vinegar
- 1/2 cup extra virgin olive oil
- 2 teaspoons garlic powder
- 2 teaspoons dried basil
- 1 teaspoon dried thyme
- 1 teaspoon dried oregano
- 1 tablespoon honey
- 1/4 teaspoon salt

Method:

1. Add vinegar, oil, and honey to a bowl a bowl. Whisk well and add dried herbs and salt. Mix well and use.

SavePrint

Mediterranean Dressing

Ingredients:

- 2 tablespoons lemon juice
- 6 tablespoons extra virgin olive oil
- 2 cloves garlic, peeled, minced
- Salt to taste
- Pepper powder to taste

Method:

1. Add all the ingredients to a bowl. Whisk well and use.

Vegan Pesto

Ingredients:

- 3/4 cup walnuts
- 3/4 cup pine nuts
- 1 1/2 cups silken tofu
- 4 cloves garlic, chopped
- 10 teaspoons white miso
- 8 cups packed basil leaves
- 4 tablespoons nutritional yeast
- 1 teaspoon ground black pepper
- 1 teaspoon sea salt
- 1 teaspoon black pepper powder

Method:

1. Add pine nuts and walnuts to the food processor and pulse for a few seconds until it is finely chopped. Add about 1/4 of the basil and pulse again. Repeat with the remaining basil.
2. Add rest of the ingredients and pulse until smooth and creamy. Chill in the refrigerator until use.

Chapter 10: Smoothie Recipes

Strawberry Smoothie

Ingredients:

- 8 large strawberries, chopped
- 1 large banana, chopped
- 2 cups fresh orange juice
- 1/2 cup low fat plain yogurt
- 2 tablespoons honey
- 2 tablespoons tahini
- 1 teaspoon vanilla extract

Method:

1. Add all the ingredients to a blender and blend until smooth.
2. Pour into tall glasses and serve with crushed ice.

Avocado Vanilla Smoothie

Ingredients:

- 2 ripe avocadoes, peeled, pitted, chopped
- 2 cups pear nectar, unsweetened or more if required
- 1 teaspoon vanilla extract

Method:

1. Add all the ingredients to a blender and blend until smooth.
2. Pour into tall glasses and serve with crushed ice.

Orange Berry Smoothie

Ingredients:

- 4 oranges, peeled, deseeded, separated into segments, skinned
- 1 1/2 cups frozen blueberries
- 1 1/2 cups frozen raspberries
- 1 1/2 cups frozen blackberries

Method:

1. Add all the ingredients to a blender and blend until smooth.
2. Pour into tall glasses and serve.

High Energy Breakfast Smoothie

Ingredients:

- 1 large banana, chopped
- 1 cup strawberries, chopped
- 5 tablespoons almond butter
- 4 tablespoons ground flaxseeds
- 3 cups low fat milk or any other milk of your choice
- 3 tablespoons blackstrap molasses

Method:

1. Add all the ingredients to a blender and blend until smooth.
2. Pour into tall glasses and serve with crushed ice.

Sunrise Surprise

Ingredients:

- 1 grapefruit, peeled, separated into segments, deseeded, skinned
- 1 orange, peeled, separated into segments, deseeded, skinned
- 4 strawberries, sliced
- 2 cups orange juice
- 2 cups grapefruit juice

Method:

1. Add all the ingredients to a blender and blend until smooth.
2. Pour into tall glasses and serve with crushed ice.

Carrot Mango Smoothie

Ingredients:

- 2 ripe mangoes, peeled, pitted, chopped into chunks or 3 cups frozen mango
- 2 cups fresh carrot juice
- A pinch grated nutmeg
- 1 small carrot, grated

Method:

1. Add all the ingredients to a blender and blend until smooth.
2. Pour into tall glasses and serve with crushed ice.

Chapter 11: Whole Foods Salad Recipes

Halibut Salad

Ingredients:

- 1 pound mixed salad greens, rinsed, pat dried
- 12 ounces halibut steaks or fillets
- 8 cloves garlic, peeled, pressed
- 2/3 cup fresh lemon juice
- 2 cups vegetable broth
- 1/3 cup fresh sage, minced or 2 tablespoons dried sage
- Salt to taste
- Pepper powder to taste
- 6 tablespoons extra virgin olive oil (optional)

Method:

1. Brush halibut steaks with lemon juice. Sprinkle salt and pepper.
2. Pour broth in a skillet and place on medium heat. Add halibut, cover and cook until done.
3. Meanwhile, divide and place the salad greens over individual serving plates.
4. Remove the halibut from the pan and place over the greens.
5. Discard the broth. To the same pan add garlic, sage and lemon juice and heat for half a minute.

6. If you are using olive oil add it after removing it from heat. Pour over the salad. Sprinkle some salt and pepper and serve.

Green Bean, Corn and Tomato Salad

Ingredients:

- 3/4 pound green beans, stringed, chopped into 1 inch pieces
- 2 cloves garlic, peeled, pressed
- 2 ears fresh corn, remove outer covering
- 1 red onion, halved, sliced
- 2 medium yellow tomatoes, sliced into 1/2 inch rounds
- 4 cups red and green heirloom tomatoes, halved
- 1/2 cup extra virgin olive oil
- 1/3 cup red wine vinegar
- Salt to taste
- Pepper powder to taste

Method:

1. Place a pot of water with some salt over medium heat. Add corn to it and boil until corn is tender. Remove from the pot and set aside to cool.
2. Add beans to the pot and cook until tender. Drain and set aside to cool.
3. When corn is cool enough to handle, remove the kernels off the cobs and place in a large bowl along with beans. Add garlic and half the oil. Toss well and set aside for about 30 minutes.
4. Remove garlic from the bowl and add rest of the ingredients. Toss well and serve.

Quinoa Salad

Ingredients:

- 1 cup quinoa
- 2 cups water
- 2 ripe, firm avocado, peeled, pitted, diced
- 2 large tomatoes, diced
- 2 -3 medium cucumbers, peeled, diced
- Salt to taste
- Pepper powder to taste
- 1/4 cup extra virgin olive oil
- 2 bunches flat leaf parsley, rinsed, chopped, discard the thick stems

Method:

1. Place a saucepan over medium heat. Add water and salt and bring to a boil.
2. Add quinoa and mix well.
3. Lower heat, cover and simmer for about 15 minutes or until the water has been absorbed.
4. Let it cool completely. Fluff with a fork and transfer into a serving dish.
5. Add rest of the ingredients. Toss well and serve.

Fattoush

Ingredients:

- 1 (6-inch) whole-wheat pita bread, split
- 1 1/2 tablespoons extra-virgin olive oil, divided
- ¾ teaspoon ground sumac, divided
- 2 tablespoons lemon juice
- 1/4 teaspoon salt or to taste
- Freshly ground pepper to taste
- 1 medium head romaine lettuce, coarsely chopped
- 1 large tomatoes, diced
- 1 small salad cucumber, diced
- ¼ cup red onions, thinly sliced
- 1 tablespoon fresh mint, thinly chopped

Method:

1. Place the pita halves on a baking sheet with the rough side up. Brush with 1/2tablespoon olive oil and sprinkle half the sumac.
2. Bake in a preheated oven at 350 degree for about 15 minutes or until crisp and golden. When cool, chop into bite size pieces.
3. In a glass bowl add lemon juice, salt, pepper, remaining oil, and sumac. Whisk well. Add rest of the ingredients and the pita pieces.
4. Toss well to coat.
5. Serve after 15 minutes.

Soy Bean and Fennel Salad

Ingredients:

- 6 cups cooked soy beans
- 16 cherry tomatoes, quartered
- 2 cups fennel bulb, sliced
- 1 large onion, minced
- 4 cloves garlic, peeled, pressed
- 1/3 cup fresh parsley, chopped
- 1/3 cup walnuts, chopped
- 1/3 cup fresh lemon juice
- 2 tablespoons extra virgin olive oil
- Salt to taste
- Pepper powder to taste

Method:

1. Add all the ingredients to a large bowl and toss well. Set aside for at least an hour before serving.

Brown Rice Salad with Apples, Walnuts, and Cherries

Ingredients:

- 2 cups brown rice
- 4 cups water
- 2 apples, diced into 1/2 inch pieces
- 1 1/2 cups frozen peas, thawed
- 2/3 cup walnuts, chopped
- 1/2 cup dried cherries, roughly chopped
- 2 bunch chives, finely chopped
  For dressing:
- 4 cloves garlic, minced
- 2 tablespoons agave syrup
- 4 tablespoons canola oil
- 1/2 cup sesame seeds, toasted
- 2 teaspoons yellow miso paste
- 4 tablespoons balsamic vinegar

Method:

1. Place rice and water in a large saucepan and cook until done. Fluff the cooked rice and cool completely.
2. Mix together rest of the ingredients in a large bowl. Add rice and toss well.
3. To make the dressing: Mix together all the ingredients of the dressing. Whisk well.
4. Pour the dressing over it and toss well and serve.

Grape and Arugula Salad

Ingredients:

- 8 cups arugula, rinsed, pat dried
- 2 cups green grapes, seedless, rinsed, pat dried
- 6-ounce Gorgonzola cheese, shredded
- 1/4 cup fresh fennel greens, rinsed, pat dried sliced
  For dressing:
- 2 tablespoons fresh lemon juice
- 2 tablespoons extra virgin olive oil
- Salt to taste
- Pepper powder to taste

Method:

1. Mix together all the ingredients of dressing and set aside.
2. Place grapes and arugula over individual serving plates.
3. Sprinkle cheese over it. Pour dressing over it and serve.

Chapter 12: Whole Food Soup Recipes

Golden Squash Soup

Ingredients:

- 2 medium sized butternut squash, peeled, deseeded, cubed
- 2 large onions, chopped
- 2 inch piece fresh ginger, peeled, minced
- 6 cloves garlic, chopped
- 6 cups vegetable broth
- 12 ounce coconut milk
- 2 teaspoons curry powder
- 1 teaspoon turmeric powder
- 1/4 cup fresh cilantro, chopped
- 1 teaspoon salt or to taste
- 1/2 teaspoon white pepper powder or to taste
- 1 tablespoon olive oil

Method:

1. Take a large saucepan and place over medium heat. Add oil. When oil is heated, add onions and sauté until translucent.
2. Add turmeric, garlic, ginger and curry powder and sauté for a couple of minutes until fragrant. Add squash and broth and bring to a boil.
3. Lower heat and simmer until tender. Remove from heat and cool slightly. Add coconut milk and blend

with an immersion blender or blend in a blender until smooth.

4. Reheat the soup. If you find the soup too thick, add some more broth, garnish with cilantro and serve.

Summer Soup

Ingredients:

- 4 cups fat free, plain yogurt
- 1 cup cilantro, chopped
- 8 large tomatoes, diced into 1 inch pieces
- 2 large red bell peppers, diced into ½ inch pieces
- 2 large cucumbers, peeled, deseeded, sliced
- 2 large onions, chopped
- 6 cups tomato juice, low sodium
- 1/2 cup red wine vinegar
- 4 teaspoons red pepper sauce or to taste
- 1/2 teaspoon black pepper powder
- 2 cloves garlic, minced

Method:

1. Mix together 1-cup yogurt and cilantro, set aside.
2. Blend together half of each tomatoes, bell pepper, cucumber, onions, and the remaining yogurt. Blend until smooth.
3. Add the tomato juice, vinegar, pepper sauce, garlic and pepper powder and blend until smooth.
4. Add the remaining half of the chopped vegetables and stir. Chill.
5. Serve into bowls topped with the cilantro – yogurt mixture.

Chicken and Brown Rice Soup

Ingredients:

- 1 large chicken breast, cut into bite sized pieces
- 3 stalks celery, chopped
- 1 large onion, chopped
- 5 medium carrots, peeled, chopped
- 1 1/2 cups long grain brown rice
- 2 bay leaves
- 2 bunches collard greens, hard ribs and stems removed, thinly sliced
- 12 cups low sodium chicken broth, divided
- 3 cups water
- Salt to taste
- Pepper powder to taste

Method:

1. Place a large pot over medium heat. Add 1/2-cup broth and bring to a boil. Add onions, carrots and celery and cook until the onions are translucent.
2. Add rest of the ingredients except collard greens and bring to a boil.
3. Lower heat, cover and cook until tender. Discard bay leaves.
4. Add collard greens and cook until collard greens wilts and serve immediately.

Mixed Mushroom Soup

Ingredients:

- 1 1/2 pounds shiitake or cremini mushrooms or a mixture of both, trimmed, chopped
- 8 ounce white button mushrooms, trimmed, chopped
- 4 shallots, chopped
- 9 cups mushroom broth or vegetable broth
- 2 teaspoons sherry vinegar
- 2 tablespoons low sodium tamari
- 1 tablespoon fresh parsley, minced
- 1 tablespoon fresh thyme

Method:

1. Retain about 1/2 pound of shiitake or cremini mushrooms and about 4 ounce of button mushrooms and add rest of it to a large pot along with shallots, broth, vinegar and tamari.
2. Place the pot over medium high heat. Bring to a boil.
3. Lower heat, cover, and cook until tender. Remove from heat and cool slightly. Blend until smooth in a blender or with an immersion blender. Add the blended soup back to the pot.
4. Add the retained mushrooms and simmer for a while until tender. Garnish with thyme and parsley and serve hot.

Kale Soup

Ingredients

- 1 large onion, chopped
- 2 carrots, peeled, cubed
- 4 red potatoes, rinsed, scrubbed, cubed
- 6 cups kale, hard ribs and stems removed, finely sliced
- 4 stalks celery, chopped
- 10 cups vegetable stock
- 4 teaspoons dried sage
- 4 teaspoons dried thyme
- Salt to taste
- Pepper powder to taste

Method:

1. Place a large saucepan over medium heat. Add about a tablespoon of broth. Add onions and sauté until onions are translucent. Add garlic and sauté for a couple of minutes.
2. Add rest of the ingredients except kale and bring to a boil.
3. Lower heat, cover and cook until tender.
4. Add kale and cook until kale wilts and serve immediately.

Chapter 13: Whole Food Snack Recipes

Grilled Pineapple

Ingredients:

- 2 cans (8 ounce each) unsweetened pineapple slices (you can use fresh pineapple slices too)
- 2 large jalapenos, seeded, minced
- Juice of 2 limes
- 1/4 teaspoon cayenne pepper
- A large pinch salt

Method:

1. Preheat a grill and grill the pineapple pieces on both the sides until brown.
2. Once cool enough to handle, chop the pineapple slices into bite-sized pieces. Transfer into a bowl.
3. Add rest of the ingredients. Mix well. Cover and refrigerate for about an hour before serving. Stir in between a couple of times.

Devilled Eggs

Ingredients:

- 3 large hard boiled eggs, cooled, shelled, halved lengthwise
- 1 tablespoon mayonnaise
- 1/2 tablespoon Dijon mustard
- 2 tablespoons parsley, minced
- 2 tablespoons diced celery, finely diced
- 1 teaspoon shallots, minced
- Celtic sea salt to taste
- Pepper powder to taste
- Paprika for garnishing

Method:

1. Remove the yolks and mash it in a bowl. Keep the whites aside.
2. Add the mayonnaise, mustard, celery, parsley, shallots, salt, and pepper. Mix well
3. Fill this mixture in the yolk portion of egg whites.
4. Refrigerate until use.
5. Sprinkle paprika and serve.

Zucchini Pizza

Ingredients:

- 3 large zucchinis, cut into ¼ inch thick round slices
- Nonstick cooking spray
- Salt to taste
- Freshly ground black pepper to taste
- 1/2 cup marinara sauce
- 1/2 cup shredded part-skim mozzarella
- 1cup tomatoes, chopped
- 1 bell pepper, chopped
- 1 large onion, sliced
- Italian seasoning to taste

Method:

1. Spray the zucchini slices with cooking spray on both the sides. Season with salt and pepper and grill on both the sides for 2 minutes per side.
2. Lay the grilled zucchini slices on a lined baking sheet.
3. Spread marinara sauce over the slices. Sprinkle onions, tomatoes and bell pepper over it. Sprinkle salt and pepper.
4. Top with cheese. Broil for a couple of minutes until the cheese is melted.

Spicy Nuts

Ingredients:

- 2 cups almonds or any nuts of your choice
- 1 tablespoon extra-virgin olive oil
- 1 1/2 teaspoon ground cumin
- 1/2teaspoon salt
- 1/2 teaspoon cayenne pepper or to taste

Method:

1. Place the almonds or nuts in a baking dish. Add all the ingredients and toss well.
2. Bake in a preheated oven at 350 degree F for about 30 minutes or until done.
3. Cool and store in an airtight container.

Zucchini/Kale Chips

Ingredients:

- 1 medium sized zucchini, sliced into about 5 mm thickness OR a bunch of kale leaves, rinsed, drained, dried, tear the leaves
- Cooking spray
- Salt to taste

Method:

1. Sprinkle salt on the zucchini or kale. Spray with cooking spray. Keep aside for a while.
2. Lay the zucchini slices on a greased baking sheet OR spread the leaves on the sheet.
3. Bake in a preheated oven at 250 degree F until crisp.

Chapter 14: Whole food Lean Meat Meal Recipes

Curried Chicken over Spinach

Ingredients:

- 2 chicken breasts, skinless, boneless, cut into bite sized pieces
- 1 cup chicken stock
- 1 medium onion, halved, sliced
- 1 small red bell pepper, thinly sliced
- 2 teaspoons fresh ginger, minced
- 2 cloves garlic, sliced
- 1/4 teaspoon turmeric powder
- 1 teaspoon curry powder
- 1/3 cup coconut milk
- 3 bunches fresh spinach, rinsed, sliced, blanched in boiling hot water for a minute
- Salt to taste
- Pepper powder to taste
- Cooking spray

Method:

1. Place a nonstick skillet over medium heat. Spray with cooking spray. Add onions and sauté until the onions are translucent. Add ginger and garlic and sauté for a couple of minutes until fragrant.
2. Add turmeric and curry powder and stir for a few seconds. Add stock, chicken and coconut milk and

cook until chicken is tender. Add bell pepper and cook for another 5 minutes.

3. Drain water remaining in the spinach. Divide and place on individual serving plates. Sprinkle salt and pepper. Serve chicken curry over it.

Chicken Taco Pizza

Ingredients:

- 2 whole wheat pizza crusts, freshly made or frozen
- 1 cup salsa – refer chapter 2 for homemade salsa or you can use store brought ones too
- 2 cups frozen corn, thawed
- 2 cups part skim mozzarella cheese, grated, divided
- 2 cups cooked black beans, rinsed, drained
- 2 frozen chicken breasts, skinless, boneless, thawed, chopped into bite sized pieces
- 1/2 cup fresh cilantro, chopped

Method:

1. Lay the pizza crusts on a large baking sheet. Divide salsa and spread over both the crusts. Sprinkle half the cheese over the salsa.
2. Sprinkle beans, corn, and chicken over the cheese. Finally, top with the remaining half cheese.
3. Bake in a preheated oven 425 degree F until the cheese is melted and slightly brown.
4. Cut into wedges and serve with some more salsa.

African Curry

Ingredients:

- 1/2 tablespoon olive oil
- 1 small onion, chopped
- 2 cloves garlic, peeled, chopped
- 1 bay leaf
- 1/2 a 14.5 ounce can whole, peeled tomatoes, drained
- 1 teaspoon curry powder
- 1/8 teaspoon salt
- 1 1/2 pound chicken, skinless, boneless, chopped into pieces
- 1/2 a 14 ounce can unsweetened coconut milk
- 1 tablespoon lemon juice

Method:

1. Place a heavy skillet over medium heat. Add oil. When oil is heated, add onion, garlic and bay leaf. Sauté for a while until the onions turn light brown.
2. Add tomatoes, curry powder, and salt. Cook for about 5 more minutes.
3. Add chicken. Mix well and cook until the chicken is tender.
4. Lower heat. Gradually add coconut milk stirring constantly. Remove from heat. Add lemon juice and serve.

Chicken & Broccoli Casserole

Ingredients:

- 30 ounces chicken breast, cooked, chopped into bite sized pieces
- 3 cups low fat Greek yogurt
- 2 cups chicken broth + extra if required
- 2 cups reduced-fat mozzarella cheese, shredded
- 2 cups cooked quinoa
- 2 cups cooked brown rice
- 4 cups fresh broccoli, chopped
- 1/2 cup red onion
- 1 cup crushed amaranth flakes,
- 1 cup wheat breadcrumbs
- 2 tablespoons Italian seasoning
- Sea salt to taste
- Pepper powder to taste

Method:

1. Mix together in a bowl the chicken, broccoli, brown rice and quinoa mix, red onions, yogurt, broth, mozzarella and Italian seasoning.
2. Transfer into a casserole dish. Spread a layer of wheat bread crumbs all over the dish. Sprinkle amaranth flakes.
3. Bake in a preheated oven at 375 degree F for about 25-30 minutes or until done.

Roast Turkey Breast with Chipotle Chili Sauce

Ingredients:

- 1 turkey breast, roasted, sliced
  For sauce:
- 1 large onion, minced
- 6 cloves garlic, minced
- 4 canned chipotle chilies, minced
- 4 tablespoons tomato paste
- 4 tablespoons Dijon mustard
- 2 cups chicken broth
- 2 tablespoons fresh oregano, chopped
- 4 tablespoons blackstrap molasses
- 1 tablespoon olive oil
- Salt to taste

Method:

1. To make sauce: Place a skillet over medium heat. Add oil. When oil is heated, add onions and sauté until onions are translucent. Add garlic and sauté until fragrant.
2. Add rest of the ingredients and simmer until thickened.
3. Serve roasted turkey with some sauce poured on it.

Turkey and Wild Rice Casserole

Ingredients:

- 1 pound turkey, cooked, shredded
- 4 cups uncooked wild rice blend
- 8 cups water
- 1 large onion, chopped
- 3 bay leaves
- 1 pound yellow squash, grated along with the skin and seeds
- 4 tablespoons olive oil, divided
- 3 tablespoons whole wheat flour
- 2 1/2 cups hot chicken broth
- 1/4 teaspoon ground nutmeg
- 3/4 cup dried cranberries
- 3/4 cup walnuts, finely chopped
- Salt to taste
- Pepper powder to taste
- 3 tablespoons fresh mixed herbs, chopped

Method:

1. Place a large pot with water over medium heat. Add rice and bay leaves and bring to a boil.
2. Lower heat, cover and cook until the rice is tender. When done, discard bay leaves and fluff rice with a fork
3. Meanwhile, place a skillet over medium heat. Add half the oil. When oil is heated, add onions and sauté until translucent. Add wheat flour and stir-fry for a couple of minutes more.
4. Add broth stirring constantly and bring to a boil.

5. Lower heat, and cook until the sauce is thick. Add nutmeg, salt and pepper and remove from heat.
6. Place another large skillet over medium high heat. Add the remaining oil. Add squash, salt and pepper. Cook until soft and transfer into a large bowl. Add the cooked wild rice, sauce and rest of the ingredients and toss well.
7. Transfer into a greased casserole dish and bake in a preheated oven at 400 degree F until the top is golden brown.

Turkey Open faced Sandwich

Ingredients:

- 4 slices multi grain sandwich bread
- 2 teaspoons Dijon style mustard
- 4 slices low sodium cooked or smoked turkey
- 2 pears, cored, thinly sliced
- 1/2 cup low fat mozzarella cheese
- Coarsely ground pepper powder to taste
- A bunch of grapes
- Few cucumber slices
- A few snap peas

Method:

1. Apply a teaspoon of mustard on each of the bread slices.
2. Place a slice of turkey on each of the bread.
3. Place pear slices over the turkey.
4. Sprinkle cheese. Finally sprinkle pepper.
5. Broil placing it 4-5 inches away from heat until the cheese melts.
6. Cut into triangles and serve.

Beef, Bean and Vegetable Chili

Ingredients:

- 1 pound 95% lean, ground beef
- 2 large onions, chopped
- 2 green bell peppers, chopped
- 2 red bell peppers, chopped
- 2 yellow bell peppers, chopped
- 3 cups frozen corn kernels
- 6 cloves garlic, finely chopped
- 4 cans (15 ounce each) unsalted kidney beans or black beans
- 1/2 cup bulgur
- 6 cups beef broth
- 1 cup water
- 1/2 cup tomato paste
- 4 tablespoons chili powder or to taste
- 2 teaspoons ground cumin
- 2 teaspoons extra virgin olive oil

Method:

1. Place a large skillet over medium high heat. Add oil. When oil is heated, add beef and cook until brown simultaneously breaking it.
2. Add onion and garlic and sauté for some more time.
3. Add rest of the ingredients. Mix well.
4. Cover and cook until bulgur is cooked. Let it remain covered at least for 15-20 minutes before serving.

Shepherd's Pie

Ingredients:

- 1 large baking potato, peeled, diced
- 1/4 cup low fat milk
- 1/2 pound lean ground beef
- 1 medium onion, chopped
- 2 cloves garlic, minced
- 1 tablespoon whole wheat flour
- 2 cups frozen mixed vegetables
- 1/2 cup low sodium beef broth
- 1/4 cup low fat cheddar cheese, sliced
- Pepper powder to taste

Method:

1. Place the potatoes in a saucepan covered with water. Cook until the potatoes are done. Drain and mash the potatoes.
2. Add milk to the mashed potatoes and mix well. Keep aside
3. Place a skillet over medium heat. Add onion, garlic, and meat. Cook until the meat is browned.
4. Add vegetables and broth. Cook until thoroughly heated.
5. Transfer to a baking dish. Spread the potato mixture over this.
6. Sprinkle cheese on top.
7. Bake in a preheated oven at 375 degree for 25 -30 minutes or until the cheese is lightly browned.

Beef Goulash with Polenta

Ingredients:

- 1 pound lean beef roast, chopped into bite sized pieces
- 1 cup polenta, uncooked
- 3 1/2 cups water
- 1 medium onion, chopped
- 2 cloves garlic, minced
- 2 tablespoons extra virgin olive oil, divided
- 1/2 a 28 ounce can whole tomatoes, crushed
- 1/2 cup low sodium chicken broth
- 1/4 cup flat leaf parsley, chopped + extra for garnishing
- 2 tablespoons Parmegiano Reggiano cheese, grated
- Sea salt to taste

Method:

1. Place a skillet over medium high heat. Add half the oil. When oil is heated, add onions and garlic and sauté until golden brown. Remove with a slotted spoon and set aside
2. Add remaining oil to the skillet. Add beef and cook until brown on all sides. Add the browned onions, tomatoes and parsley and mix well.
3. Lower heat, cover and cook until beef is tender.
4. Uncover and cook for another 30 minutes. Simultaneously, add water to a medium pot and place over medium heat. Add salt and polenta gently stirring constantly.

5. Lower heat and cook until the polenta is done and comes off from the sides of the pot.
6. Serve beef over polenta. Garnish with cheese and parsley and serve hot.

Chapter 15: Whole Foods Seafood Recipes

Baked Halibut

Ingredients:

- 3 pounds halibut steak or fillet chopped into pieces
- 6 cloves garlic, peeled, pressed
- 1/2 cup chicken broth
- 1/4 cup capers
- 1/4 cup lemon juice
- 1/4 cup fresh parsley, chopped
- 2 tablespoons fresh chives, chopped
- 2 tablespoons fresh tarragon, chopped
- Salt to taste
- Pepper powder to taste

Method:

1. Place halibut in a greased baking dish. Add rest of the ingredients. Toss well.
2. Bake in a preheated oven at 450 degree F for about 15-20 minutes or until done.
3. Serve immediately.

Caribbean Seafood Stew

Ingredients:

- 1/2 pound shrimp
- 1/2 pound mahi-mahi fish, chopped into pieces
- 1 yellow onions, chopped
- 3 cloves garlic, minced
- 1 tablespoon ground cumin
- 2 tablespoons cilantro, chopped
- 2 tomatoes, chopped
- 1/2 can coconut milk
- 1/2 tablespoon coconut oil
- Sea salt to taste
- Pepper powder to taste

Method:

1. Place a saucepan over medium heat. Add coconut oil. When the oil heats up, add onions. Sauté for 3-4 minutes, Add garlic and cilantro and sauté for 2-3 minutes.
2. Add the tomatoes, cumin, salt and pepper. Sauté for a couple of minutes more.
3. Reduce heat and add coconut milk, shrimps and mahi-mahi. Simmer for 5-7 minutes or until the fish is flaky.
4. Garnish with cilantro and serve.

Wild Salmon with Lentils and Arugula

Ingredients:

- 1 1/2 cups green lentils
- 6 fillets (6 ounce each) wild salmon, skinless
- 5 cups baby arugula
- 2 stalks celery, chopped
- 2 carrots, peeled, diced
- 1 large onion, chopped
- 2 bay leaves
- 3 tablespoons extra virgin olive oil + extra for drizzling
- 2 tablespoons lemon juice
- Sea salt to taste
- Pepper powder to taste

Method:

1. Add onions, carrots, celery, bay leaf and lentils to a large pot and place it over medium heat. Bring to a boil.
2. Lower heat, cover and cook until tender. Drain and set aside. Add salt, pepper, oil and lemon juice,
3. Add arugula, mix well, cover and keep aside.
4. Place the fillets in a baking dish. Drizzle olive oil, sprinkle salt and pepper. Cover with aluminum foil.
5. Bake in a preheated oven at 375 degree F until done.
6. Serve with lentils. Sprinkle lemon juice on top and serve.

Peanut Shrimp

Ingredients:

- 1 pound medium size shrimp, peeled, deveined
- 1/2 cup peanut sauce of your choice or refer chapter 2
- 4 cloves garlic, chopped
- 1/2 cup fresh lemon juice
- 1/3 cup low sodium chicken or vegetable broth
- 1/4 cup extra virgin olive oil
- Salt to taste
- Pepper powder to taste
- Mixed greens to serve

Method:

1. Take about 1/3 cup lemon juice and add salt and pepper to it. Mix well and rub it over the shrimp. Set aside for about 10 minutes.
2. Place a skillet over medium low heat. Add broth and heat. Add shrimp, and cook for 2 minutes. Add garlic and cook for a couple of minutes until the shrimp turn opaque. Do not overcook, as they tend to become hard.
3. Remove from heat and drizzle oil and the remaining lemon juice.
4. Serve over mixed greens with a large dollop of peanut sauce.

Sweet N' Sour Cod with Cabbage and Broccoli

Ingredients:

- 2 pounds cod fillet, chopped into 1 inch pieces
- 1 medium onion, sliced
- 4 cups broccoli florets, cut into small florets, discard stem
- 8 cups cabbage, finely shredded
- 8 cloves garlic, peeled, pressed
- 2 tablespoons chicken or vegetable broth
- 2 tablespoons sesame seeds
- 1/4 cup fresh cilantro, chopped
- Salt to taste
- Pepper powder to taste

    For sweet n sour sauce:

- 1/2 cup rice vinegar
- 1/2 cup mirin rice vinegar
- 4 tablespoons chicken or vegetable broth
- 4 tablespoons honey
- Salt to taste
- Pepper powder to taste

Method:

1. To make sauce: Add all the ingredients to a saucepan. Mix well and place over medium heat. Simmer until the sauce thickens. Set aside.
2. Add all the ingredients except cabbage, cilantro, and sesame seeds to a skillet and place over

medium heat. Simmer for about 5 minutes. Add cabbage and simmer for a couple of minutes. Stir constantly.

3. Add the prepared sauce and cilantro and stir well.
4. Garnish with sesame seeds and serve.

Chapter 16: Whole Foods Vegetarian Meal Recipes

Curried Mustard Greens & Garbanzo Beans with Sweet Potatoes

Ingredients:

- 4 medium sweet potatoes, peeled, thinly sliced, steamed
- 2 bunches mustard greens, discard stems, chopped
- 4 cups cooked garbanzo beans, drained
- 1 large onion, halved, thinly sliced
- 6 cloves garlic, sliced
- 2 large ripe tomatoes, chopped
- 1 teaspoon curry powder
- 1/2 teaspoon turmeric powder
- 6 tablespoons extra virgin olive oil
- 3/4 cup vegetable broth
- Salt to taste
- Pepper powder to taste
- Cooking spray

Method:

1. Place a skillet over medium heat. Spray with cooking spray. Add onion and sauté until onions are translucent. Add garlic, and sauté for a few seconds until fragrant. Add curry powder, turmeric and stir-fry for a few seconds.

2. Add mustard greens and cook until the greens wilt. Add garbanzo beans, tomatoes, salt, and pepper and simmer for 5-7 minutes.
3. Meanwhile mash sweet potatoes along with broth, oil, salt and pepper.
4. Serve mustard greens on individual plates. Top with mashed sweet potato mixture and serve.

Mushroom Alfredo

Ingredients:

- 16 ounces whole wheat spelt rotini or any other whole wheat pasta, cooked according to instructions on the package
- 1 pound mixed mushrooms, trimmed, sliced
- 4 tablespoons extra virgin olive oil
- 8 cloves garlic, minced
- 14 tablespoons almonds, sliced, divided
- 1 1/2 cups almond milk, unsweetened
- 1 1/2 teaspoons fine sea salt, divided
- 1 teaspoon freshly ground black pepper powder
- 4 tablespoons nutritional yeast
- 1/4 cup fresh parsley, chopped

Method:

1. Place a large deep skillet or wok over medium high heat. Add oil. When oil is heated, add mushrooms and about a teaspoon salt. Sauté until brown.
2. Add garlic and sauté until fragrant.
3. Meanwhile toast half the almonds and set aside. Add the remaining almonds to a blender and blend along with nutritional yeast and almond milk until smooth and creamy. Add this to the skillet of mushroom.
4. Add the cooked pasta, salt and pepper to the skillet and toss well.
5. Garnish with toasted almonds and parsley and serve.

Moroccan Eggplant with Garbanzo Beans

Ingredients:

- 1 large eggplant, chopped into 1 inch cubes
- 1 red bell pepper, chopped into 1 inch squares
- 1 green bell pepper, chopped into 1 inch squared
- 2 large onions, halved, sliced
- 10 cloves garlic, peeled, pressed
- 1 teaspoon turmeric
- 1 teaspoon Moroccan spice blend
- 2 cans (15 ounce each) lentils, drained
- 4 cups canned or home cooked garbanzo beans drained
- 1 cup tomato sauce
- 2 3/4 cups vegetable broth
- 1 cup raisins
- 1 teaspoon red chili flakes or to taste
- Salt to taste
- Pepper powder to taste
- 2 tablespoons freshly chopped cilantro

Method:

1. Add about 2 tablespoons of broth to a large skillet. Place the skillet over medium heat. Add onions and cook for about 5 minutes. Add garlic, bell peppers, eggplant, spice blend and turmeric. Sauté for a couple of minutes. Add remaining broth and tomato sauce.
2. Lower heat; simmer until the eggplants are tender. Stir in between a couple of times. Add rest of the

ingredients except cilantro, stir and simmer for 5-7 minutes.

3. Garnish with cilantro and serve.

Creamy Risotto with Butternut Squash

Ingredients:

- 2 cups raw cashews, soaked in water overnight, drained
- 5 cups butternut squash, peeled, deseeded, chopped
- 2 packages (20 ounce each) frozen brown rice
- 1 cup onion, chopped
- 6 cloves garlic, minced
- 1/2 cup fresh parsley, finely chopped
- 3 cups non-dairy milk like soy milk or almond milk
- 1 teaspoon fine sea salt
- 1 teaspoon ground cinnamon
- 1 1/2 cups low sodium vegetable broth
- 4 tablespoons fresh sage, minced
- 1/2 teaspoon freshly ground black pepper
- Cooking spray

Method:

1. Place a large pot over medium heat. Add squash and cook until tender. Remove about 1 1/2 cups of the squash and keep it aside.
2. Let the rest of the squash cook for another 10 minutes or until very soft. Drain and set aside.
3. Meanwhile, blend together in a blender, cashew, softened squash, milk, cinnamon and salt until smooth and creamy. Set it aside.
4. Place a large skillet over medium heat. Spray with cooking spray. Add onions and garlic and sauté until light brown.

5. Add the cup of squash that was kept aside, brown rice and broth. Cook for 2-3 minutes stirring on and off.

6. Add creamy cashew mixture, sage and parsley. Stir and lower heat. Simmer until risotto of the desired thickness is achieved.

7. Remove from heat. Sprinkle black pepper powder and stir. Serve hot.

Greek Style Quinoa Burgers

Ingredients:

- 1 cup quinoa, rinsed
- 1 1/2 cups water
- 1 large carrots, peeled, roughly chopped
- 12 scallions, thinly sliced, divided
- 1/2 cup whole wheat dried bread crumbs
- 2 cans (15 ounce each) Great northern beans, drained, rinsed
- 2 tablespoons ground cumin
- Salt to taste
- Pepper powder to taste
- 1 cup non fat, plain Greek yogurt
- 1 English cucumber, thinly sliced, diagonally
- 2 tablespoons lemon juice
- 4 tablespoons olive oil
- 8 pitas (6 inches each)

Method:

1. Place a saucepan over medium heat. Add water and bring to a boil. Add quinoa, stir and lower heat. Cook until quinoa is tender and water is almost dried up. Keep it aside to cool.
2. Add carrots to the food processor and pulse for a few seconds until it is finely chopped. Add quinoa, half the scallions, beans, breadcrumbs, cumin powder, salt, and pepper and pulse until well combined. The beans need not be finely mashed.
3. Remove the mixture from the food processor and form into 8 patties of about 3/4 inch thick.

4. Place a nonstick pan over medium heat. Cook the patties in batches. Add half the oil. Place 3-4 patties and cook until brown on both the sides.
5. Add the remaining oil and cook rest of the patties.
6. Meanwhile mix together in a bowl, yogurt, lemon juice, remaining scallions, salt and pepper.
7. Place the patties in the pita. Top with yogurt sauce and cucumber.

Chapter 17: Whole Food Side Dishes Recipes

Fennel Green Beans

Ingredients:

- 6 cups thin green beans, stringed, chopped into 1 inch pieces, steamed
- 1 medium onion, sliced
- 1 cup fennel bulb, sliced
- 2 fresh tomatoes, deseeded, chopped
- 2 tablespoons extra virgin olive oil
- 4 tablespoons fresh lemon juice
- Salt to taste
- Pepper powder to taste
- Cooking spray

Method:

1. Place a skillet over medium heat. Spray with cooking spray. Add onions and sauté until translucent. Add fennel and sauté for a couple of minutes.
2. Add beans and rest of the ingredients. Toss well and serve.

Mashed Potatoes with Garlic

Ingredients:

- 4 large potatoes, peeled, cubed, steamed
- ½ cup low fat milk or any other nondairy milk of your choice
- ½ cup extra-virgin olive oil
- 6 cloves garlic, minced
- Sea salt to taste
- Pepper powder to taste

Method:

1. Mash hot, steamed potatoes in a large bowl. Add rest of the ingredients and mix well.

Roasted Cauliflower Steaks

Ingredients:

- 2 heads cauliflower, stems removed, rinsed
- 4 cloves garlic, crushed
- 2 tablespoons lemon juice
- ¼ cup fresh parsley

Method:

1. Mix together lemon juice and garlic in a bowl and set it aside for a while.
2. Hold the cauliflower on your cutting board and start slicing it into ¾ inch thick slices (do not separate florets in this recipe)
3. Place the cauliflower slices on a lined baking sheet. Brush the slices with lemon juice and place the garlic on the baking sheet.
4. Roast in a preheated oven at 375 degree F until golden brown.
5. Garnish with parsley and serve.

Baked Root Vegetables

Ingredients:

- 8 medium potatoes, washed, cut into cubes
- 1 large sweet potato, scrubbed, washed, cut into cubes
- 1 carrot, scrubbed, washed, cut into cubes
- 1 beetroot, peeled, cut into cubes
- 1 turnip, peeled, cut into cubes
- 2 tablespoons lemon juice
- 200 g yam, peeled, cut into cubes
- 1 cup water
- 2 tablespoons dill, chopped
- Pepper powder to taste

Method:

1. Place the root vegetables in a glass-baking dish.
2. Add water. Cover the dish with a foil. Prick the foil at a couple of places with a fork.
3. Bake in preheated oven at 400 degree F for about 45 minutes.
4. Remove from oven. Sprinkle lemon juice and dill. Toss well to coat.
5. Serve hot.

Beef and Green Bean Stir Fry

Ingredients:

- 1/2 pound lean steak, cut into cubes
- 1 cup fresh green beans, stringed, cut into 2 inch pieces, blanched
- 1 small onion, thinly sliced
- 1 small red bell pepper, thinly sliced
- 2 cloves garlic, minced
- 2 tablespoon tamari or soy sauce
- 2 tablespoons white wine
- 1 tablespoon peanut oil, divided
- 2 teaspoons honey
- 2 teaspoons arrowroot powder
- Sea salt to taste
- Pepper powder to taste

Method:

1. Mix together in a bowl, tamari, wine, honey and garlic. Add steak and toss well. Cover and place in the refrigerator for 3-4 hours.
2. Place a wok over medium high heat. Add half the oil. When oil is heated, add only the steak and retain the sauce mixture.
3. Sauté until the steak is cooked. Remove from the skillet and set aside.
4. Add the remaining oil to the skillet. Add onion, bell pepper and beans. Sauté for a couple of minutes. Add the cooked steak and sauté for a minute.

5. To the cooled reserved sauce, add arrowroot powder and mix until smooth. Pour this into the skillet stirring constantly until the steak and vegetables are well coated and thickened. Add salt and pepper.

Chapter 18: Whole Foods Dessert Recipes

Fresh Berries with Yogurt and Chocolate

Ingredients:

- 1 basket fresh strawberries
- 1 basket fresh raspberries
- 16 ounce low fat vanilla yogurt
- 4 ounce dark chocolate, melted in a double boiler

Method:

1. Mix berries in a large bowl. Add yogurt and fold gently.
2. Serve berries along with yogurt in individual bowls. Drizzle melted chocolate over it and serve.

Healthy Sundaes

Ingredients:

- 2 ripe bananas, sliced
- 2/3 cup pineapple, chopped
- 2/3 cup kiwi, chopped
- 4 strawberries, chopped
- 4 dates, pitted, chopped
- ¼ cup granola
- 1/3 cup boiling water
- 1/4 cup almond milk
- ¼ teaspoon ground ginger
- 1 ½ tablespoons almond butter, unsweetened

Method:

1. Soak dates in boiling water for at least 45 minutes.
2. Place banana slices on a baking sheet that is lined with parchment paper. Do not overlap the banana slices. Place the baking sheet in the freezer until the slices are frozen
3. Meanwhile blend together dates and ginger along with water into a smooth sauce and keep it aside.
4. Clean the blender and blend together the frozen bananas, almond butter and almond milk. Transfer into individual freezer safe bowls and freeze until done.
5. Remove from the freezer and sprinkle pineapple, kiwi and strawberry pieces over it. Sprinkle granola. Pour date sauce on top and serve.

Puffed Quinoa Peanut Butter Balls

Ingredients:

- 2 cups puffed quinoa
- 1 cup peanut butter
- ½ cup agave nectar
- 2 tablespoons crushed peanuts
- 2 teaspoons vanilla extract
- Dark chocolate (optional)

Method:

1. Mix together in a heatproof bowl, peanut butter, agave and vanilla. Place the bowl in a double boiler for a while until the ingredients are softened and smooth flowing.
2. Remove from heat and add puffed quinoa. Mix well and refrigerate for 15-20 minutes.
3. Remove from the refrigerator and form small balls. Dip into dark chocolate if desired. Refrigerate again for 15 minutes before serving.

Blueberry Peach Crisp

Ingredients:

- 8 blueberries, fresh or frozen (if frozen, thawed)
- 1/2 pound peach slices, fresh or frozen (if frozen, thawed)
- 2 tablespoons apple juice
  For topping:
- 1/4 cup rolled oats
- 1/4 cup almonds
- 1/2 cup dates, pitted
- 1 tablespoon apple juice
- 1/4 teaspoon ground cinnamon

Method:

1. Lay the blueberries at the bottom of a baking dish. Lay the peach slices over the blueberries. Sprinkle apple juice over it.
2. Blend together in a blender, almonds, dates, oats and cinnamon for a few seconds. Add apple juice and pulse for a few seconds.
3. Spread this mixture over the fruits in the baking dish.
4. Bake for about 45 minutes or until the top is crispy.
5. Serve either warm or cold.

Strawberry Mousse

Ingredients:

- 1 ½ pounds fresh strawberries, or 1 ½ package frozen and very well drained
- 3 tablespoons lemon juice
- Natural sweetener to taste like honey or stevia or agave nectar
- 1 teaspoon vanilla (optional)
- ½ cup coconut oil, softened
- ½ cup coconut butter, softened
- A few strawberry slices to garnish

Method:

1. Add all the ingredients to a blender and blend until smooth.
2. Pour into individual dessert bowls. Chill and serve.

Coconut and Chia Seed Pudding

Ingredients:

- 1/2 cup shredded, unsweetened coconut
- 1/2 cup chia seeds
- 1 1/2 cups full fat coconut milk
- 1 cup coconut water
- 2 teaspoons pure vanilla extract
- 1/2 teaspoon salt
- 1 cup fresh raspberries

Method:

1. In a bowl, mix together all the ingredients. Mix well.
2. Pour into serving bowls and refrigerate.
3. Serve chilled with fresh raspberries.

Conclusion

With this, we come to the end of this book. Through the course of this book, I have helped you with the benefits of this diet and also some amazing recipes that will help you cook some delicious and nutritious meals for your loved ones.

I want to thank you for choosing this book and hope you find it helpful in changing your nutrition choices in life.

Made in the USA
San Bernardino, CA
06 February 2017